D0898325

# The Minerals You Need

-Roger Mason

A complete and unique guide to all the minerals
necessary for better health and longer life

YOUNG AGAIN PRODUCTS, INC.
310 N. FRONT ST. #150
WILMINGTON, NC 28401
WWW.YOUNGAGAIN.COM
WWW.YOUNGAGAIN.ORG

# *The Minerals You Need*
by Roger Mason

Copyright© 2003 by Roger Mason
All Rights Reserved

ISBN 1-884820-75-1

Printed in the USA

Safe Goods
561 Shunpike Road
Sheffield, MA  01257
413-229-7935
www.safegoodspub.com

# CONTENTS

# About This Book

My previous five books – *The Natural Prostate Cure, Zen Macrobiotics for Americans, What is Beta Glucan?, No More Horse Estrogen!* and *Lower Cholesterol Without Drugs*- were all very heavily documented with published international studies from the most prominent scientific journals. The next two books, *Testosterone Is Your Friend* and *The Natural Diabetes Cure* will also be. In this book there is, instead, is a partial list of the many dozens of studies used. Your author went through *Chemical Abstracts* (the "Scientist's Bible") last fifteen years of research on all these minerals. Everything you read here comes directly from the world's published clinical research. You will find unique information here that's not found in other books or articles.

There are only ten minerals with an established RDA (Recommended Daily Allowance), yet we know of at least that many more that are known to be essential. There are still others that may well prove to be essential, even in the small amounts that are found in our foods and soils. There is usually a lag of many years between scientific discovery and application, in the everyday world we live in. Science has known for a long time we need to fortify both our soils and domestic animals with a variety of minerals, so that our foods will be nutritious, rather than mineral-deficient. **Science has known for a long time that lack of trace elements is responsible in part for EVERY disease, condition, and illness known to man.** Supplementing our diets with these vital minerals will go a long way towards preventing and curing the endless list of health problems we suffer from. We live in the richest, most affluent and productive country on earth, but ironically suffer from the poorest health, generally.

Why is it that farmers are not using more minerals in their soils to get better, more bountiful and more nutritious, disease-resistant crops? Why aren't ranchers giving more minerals to their livestock for healthier, more feed-efficient, and more prolific animals? Most of all, why aren't people demanding real, effective nutritional supplements with all the known minerals we need?

Please read this book so you'll know the minerals you need to be in the best of health and live a long, happy life.

VIII

# Periodic Table of the Elements

Legend:
- 6 Atomic number
- C Symbol
- 12.01 Atomic weight

| 1 | 2 | 3 | 4 | 5 | 6 | 7 | 8 | 9 | 10 | 11 | 12 | 13 | 14 | 15 | 16 | 17 | 18 |
|---|---|---|---|---|---|---|---|---|----|----|----|----|----|----|----|----|----|
| 1 **H** 1.008 | | | | | | | | | | | | | | | | | 2 **He** 4.003 |
| 3 **Li** 6.941 | 4 **Be** 9.012 | | | | | | | | | | | 5 **B** 10.81 | 6 **C** 12.01 | 7 **N** 14.01 | 8 **O** 16.00 | 9 **F** 19.00 | 10 **Ne** 20.18 |
| 11 **Na** 22.99 | 12 **Mg** 24.31 | | | | | | | | | | | 13 **Al** 26.98 | 14 **Si** 28.09 | 15 **P** 30.97 | 16 **S** 32.07 | 17 **Cl** 35.45 | 18 **Ar** 39.95 |
| 19 **K** 39.10 | 20 **Ca** 40.08 | 21 **Sc** 44.96 | 22 **Ti** 47.88 | 23 **V** 50.94 | 24 **Cr** 52.00 | 25 **Mn** 54.94 | 26 **Fe** 55.85 | 27 **Co** 58.93 | 28 **Ni** 58.69 | 29 **Cu** 63.55 | 30 **Zn** 65.39 | 31 **Ga** 69.72 | 32 **Ge** 72.61 | 33 **As** 74.92 | 34 **Se** 78.96 | 35 **Br** 79.90 | 36 **Kr** 83.80 |
| 37 **Rb** 85.47 | 38 **Sr** 87.62 | 39 **Y** 88.91 | 40 **Zr** 91.22 | 41 **Nb** 92.91 | 42 **Mo** 95.94 | 43 **Tc** 98.91 | 44 **Ru** 101.1 | 45 **Rh** 102.9 | 46 **Pd** 106.4 | 47 **Ag** 107.9 | 48 **Cd** 112.4 | 49 **In** 114.8 | 50 **Sn** 118.7 | 51 **Sb** 121.8 | 52 **Te** 127.6 | 53 **I** 126.9 | 54 **Xe** 131.3 |
| 55 **Cs** 132.9 | 56 **Ba** 137.3 | * 71 **Lu** 175.0 | 72 **Hf** 178.5 | 73 **Ta** 180.9 | 74 **W** 183.8 | 75 **Re** 186.2 | 76 **Os** 190.2 | 77 **Ir** 192.2 | 78 **Pt** 195.1 | 79 **Au** 197.0 | 80 **Hg** 200.6 | 81 **Tl** 204.4 | 82 **Pb** 207.2 | 83 **Bi** 209.0 | 84 **Po** 209.0 | 85 **At** 210.0 | 86 **Rn** 222.0 |
| 87 **Fr** 223.0 | 88 **Ra** 226.0 | ** 103 **Lr** 260.1 | 104 **Rf** 261.1 | 105 **Db** 262.1 | 106 **Sg** 263.1 | 107 **Bh** 262.1 | 108 **Hs** | 109 **Mt** | 110 **Uun** | 111 **Uuu** | 112 **Uub** | 113 **Uut** | 114 **Uuq** | 115 **Uup** | 116 **Uuh** | 117 **Uus** | 118 **Uuo** |

| 6 * | 57 **La** 136.9 | 58 **Ce** 140.1 | 59 **Pr** 140.9 | 60 **Nd** 144.2 | 61 **Pm** 146.9 | 62 **Sm** 150.4 | 63 **Eu** 152.0 | 64 **Gd** 157.3 | 65 **Tb** 158.9 | 66 **Dy** 162.5 | 67 **Ho** 164.9 | 68 **Er** 167.3 | 69 **Tm** 168.9 | 70 **Yb** 173.0 |
|---|---|---|---|---|---|---|---|---|---|---|---|---|---|---|
| 7 ** | 89 **Ac** 227.0 | 90 **Th** 232.0 | 91 **Pa** 231.0 | 92 **U** 236.0 | 93 **Np** 237.0 | 94 **Pu** 244.1 | 95 **Am** 243.1 | 96 **Cm** 247.1 | 97 **Bk** 247.1 | 98 **Cf** 251.1 | 99 **Es** 252.0 | 100 **Fm** 257.1 | 101 **Md** 258.1 | 102 **No** 259.1 |

# Chapter 1: Minerals in General

Ninety-six natural elements exist; but there are only ten with an established Recommended Daily Allowance (RDA). Those include calcium, magnesium, iron, zinc, manganese, copper, iodine, chromium, selenium and molybdenum. There are at least eight more that are known to be needed in human nutrition, with no RDA set. It is well known, for example, that boron is necessary for life, but no RDA has been set for it at this point. Just recently, it has become well known that vanadium is also necessary for life, but it is difficult to even find any vanadium in a vitamin/mineral supplement. There is no doubt silicon is a necessary mineral, but you will rarely find it offered in any supplement. There is good initial evidence that such other minerals as barium, beryllium, cesium, europium, indium, gallium, lanthanum, lithium, neodymium, praseodymium, rubidium, samarium, scandium, thulium, yttrium and other ultratrace minerals may also well be necessary for plant and animal life, if only in small daily microgram amounts of less than one-tenth of one milligram.

We basically just do not show any deficiencies of phosphorous, potassium, sodium, sulfur, chloride or fluoride. These are often used as "filler" in promotional vitamin mineral supplements.

If there is one thing to understand it is that **all minerals work together as a biological team,** just like a sports team. When one mineral is deficient, the others simply cannot do their jobs well. It is important to get all the known minerals we need, in the necessary biological amounts. Minerals often work together in pairs, synergistically. There are a few relationships we do know, such as the calcium-to-magnesium ratio and the zinc-to-copper ratio, but there are countless more relationships we have no idea of yet, and have not discovered.

Americans are overfed and undernourished. We eat twice the calories we need, from refined and devalued foods. We eat an amazing eight times the fat we need – 42 percent of our caloric intake – and most all of this is saturated animal fat. We eat twice the protein we need. We eat an unbelievable 160 pounds of various simple sugars we do not need at all. Yet we still don't get the vitamins and minerals we need in our daily food! The wealthiest country in the world is also the most mineral deficient of all. America leads the world in obesity, coronary and heart disease, blood sugar disorders, including insulin resistance and diabetes, arthritis and rheumatism, osteoporosis, PMS and menstrual problems, menopausal conditions, most types of cancer, especially prostate, breast, lung, ovarian, cervical and uterine, and most every other illness that plagues human beings.

The question comes up about which forms of the minerals to take. The various bioavailable forms of each mineral will be mentioned in following chapters. Some are inexpensive common salts such as zinc sulfate, while others are chelates (KEE-lates), which are simply minerals bound in a manner they can easily be digested. Should you take your minerals before meals, during meals, or after meals? It just doesn't matter. The important thing is that you take them every day for the rest of your life, and get all the ones you need in the biologically-required amounts.

Due to highly sophisticated analytical techniques such as PIXE, SRFXA, ANN, ICP-AES, and ICP-MS, we can now pinpoint minerals down to picograms- trillionths of a gram. (There are one million picograms in a microgram!) We can now easily and accurately measure the precise mineral content in our soils, the food we eat, our bodies, and all important actual blood levels. It would be wonderful if we could just go to the doctors office and get our blood analyzed for dozens of different vital minerals, so we can know which ones we are deficient in. We could also test the toxic, harmful ones – lead, aluminum, cadmium, mercury, and others. This is costly and, currently, we can only practically and inexpensively test a few like iron, calcium and magnesium. Urine analysis only tells us what we excrete, and not what we retain in our blood. Hair analysis is more suited for revealing harmful minerals, like arsenic poisoning. In the next 20 years the price for patient testing will come down and we will be able to measure all our basic mineral's level inexpensively.

No matter how well you eat, how many other supplements you take, how much you exercise, or anything else, you are never going to have the health you want unless you have all the vital minerals you need. Mineral nutrition still is not well understood, and the mineral supplements available are woefully incomplete.

# Chapter 2: Where Can I Find A Good Mineral Supplement?

It is simply unbelievable that it is almost impossible to find a complete mineral or vitamin/mineral supplement anywhere in the world, in the year 2004. Look in the biggest vitamin catalogs and see what kind of mineral supplements they offer – or don't offer!

Now look in any health food stores and drug stores, especially the mega-chain stores, and see if you can find a good mineral supplement. Go to the Internet and you'll see almost nothing but promotions with very poor products. What you find will be woefully incomplete and lacking not only in the minerals themselves, but, in the biological amounts you need of them.

The key to finding a valid mineral supplement is to READ THE LABEL. If it's not on the label, it's not in the bottle. You must see all the minerals listed and the exact amount contained in each tablet or capsule. If the manufacturer hides behind the loophole phrase "proprietary formula", put it back on the shelf, as there is nothing in there. Don't settle for one that contains a mere dozen minerals, even if they are in the biological amounts you need. Also, do not be taken in by "window dressing", such as potassium, sodium, phosphorous, sulfur, chloride, fluoride, and other minerals that are not needed. Adding these just makes the label *appear* better and more complete.

The biggest fraud to ever hit the natural health industry was colloidal minerals – that's until coral calcium came along a few years later. Millions of people were taken in by the most asinine claims and assertions. Pyramid schemes sold these by passing out audio tapes. If you ever read the label on a bottle of colloidal minerals, you noticed that dozens and dozens of minerals were listed, but never the AMOUNTS. Obviously, that's because there was almost nothing of any biological value in there. Merely containing meaningless amounts, such as one microgram of a certain mineral, gave them the legal right to list it on the label. You could drink a whole bottle of colloidal minerals every day and not get any benefit, except for two or three minerals at most. Fortunately this has faded into obscurity, except for some Internet advertisements.

Coral calcium succeeded colloidal minerals in the honor of being the biggest fraud in the natural health industry. This is just plain old calcium carbonate (as in blackboard chalk) with a high price tag. They also claim to have dozens and dozens of minerals contained in the formula, but the facts are it is just cheap calcium carbonate with one or two other minerals.

Why won't the largest pharmaceutical and vitamin companies in the world put out a good mineral supplement that has all the minerals we need, in the biologically required amounts? Don't these companies have extensive research facilities to develop cutting-edge products? Not at all. They have extensive ADVERTISING departments to promote second-rate products with very little actual benefits. These corporations spend almost nothing on research and development, but millions on advertising.

Look at the best-selling and most popular mineral and vitamin/mineral formulations in the world. READ THE LABEL. You'll rarely find boron, vanadium, or silicon at all, and substandard amounts of selenium, chromium, and molybdenum, even in their premier, top-of-the-line formulas. You'll never find realistic amounts of such important minerals as germanium, tin, nickel, strontium, or cobalt.

You will sometimes hear that only liquid or encapsulated supplements work, and that tablets and caplets do not dissolve in your stomach, but merely pass through your digestive system intact. This is merely advertising gimmickry. You can prove this to yourself by putting any tablet in a glass of warm water with a tablespoon of vinegar and watching it dissolve in a few hours. The human stomach is much more acidic, much warmer, and subject to a lot of physical motion, so tablets will dissolve much better in your body. You can also prove this by taking a dozen tablets of a certain product and watching your stool the next day. You will not find them in your stool as all tablets have a dissolving agent added to them at time of their manufacture.

You will also hear a lot of talk about how only a certain salt or form of a vitamin or mineral is actually bio-available. Of course it always turns out that the company saying this has a patented form of this supplement that no one else can use without paying a royalty. The absorbable forms of each mineral you need are discussed in each chapter.

# Chapter 3: Calcium

Calcium is number 20 on the Periodic Table, the fifth most abundant element, and was discovered in 1808. It has an atomic weight of 40.0, so it is a light mineral and toxicity is unknown. The RDA for calcium, in adults, is set at 1,000 mg a day. Calcium is the most abundant mineral in our bodies by far, because 99 percent of it is in our bones. Calcium carbonate, citrate, and other forms are very bio-available and inexpensive. However, being the most abundant mineral just does not make it the most important mineral.

To my way of thinking, the government-established daily allowance (RDA) is very scientifically incorrect. Asians, Africans, Mideasterners, and Latins eat a fraction of what Europeans (and Indians) eat. Dairy products are not eaten as a normal staple for the people in these countries, and although they take in less than 400mg of calcium every day at most they have far less bone and join disease than do Europeans The RDA is simply Eurocentric and can only be met by eating large amounts of milk and dairy products. Of the six billion people on earth only about one billion regularly eat dairy products as a staple food. People of all races stop secreting lactase (the enzyme that digests lactose, or milk sugar) at about the age of three. All adults, therefore, are lactose intolerant and should not drink milk or eat dairy products. Most dairy foods, like milk, cream, cheese, cream cheese, and sour cream are very high in saturated fats, and not good food choices anyway. The **only** abundant dietary source of calcium (other than sea vegetables) is dairy food; no other food group contains nearly as much.

If we look at any list of the calcium content of common foods we eat we find that other than dairy products, there is very little calcium in whole grains, beans, vegetables, fruits, seafood, or meat. To demonstrate how little calcium there is in *all* other foods, other than dairy, let's look at a generous and varied sample daily menu. If your daily diet consisted of the following you would actually ingest less than 400 mg of calcium: three cups of brown rice, two cups of oatmeal, one cup of dried beans, a cup of a green vegetable, eight ounces of fish, eight ounces of beef, a salad with dressing, four slices of whole grain bread, four pieces of fresh fruit and a cup of vegetable soup.

The research on calcium is simply overdone. Calcium is the most popular of all mineral supplements because people are led to believe they are deficient in it. The problem, however, is NOT deficient dietary calcium at all – it is the lack of ABSORPTION.

Western people take in more calcium by far than anyone else yet, have the highest rate of bone and joint disease in the world, especially arthritis and osteoporosis. The Asian, African, Mideast and Latin cultures which take in the least amount of calcium, generally have far stronger bones and joints, and far less arthritis, osteoporosis and other conditions. These people do not and cannot get anywhere near the official U.S. government recommendation of 1,000 mg every day from their diets of meat, fish, poultry, eggs, grains, vegetables, beans, and fruit. True vegetarians who don't eat dairy products also have less bone and joint conditions. The fact that five billion people eat a fraction of the suggested RDA of calcium and have far less bone and joint disease is inarguable, real world proof we just don't need 1,000 mg per day.

Taking ten grams of calcium a day isn't going to make your bones any stronger, unless you also get sufficient amounts of magnesium, boron, strontium and vitamin D. These are just the four major synergists we know of, but there are others which play smaller roles such as manganese, zinc, and silicon. Calcium just cannot work by itself to make new bone cells (osteoblasts). The fact is that we need less calcium after the age of eighteen, when our skeletons are fully formed. As we age, we need less calories and less calcium than when we were younger. To have strong bones and avoid arthritis and osteoporosis, we have to take in ALL the known minerals to work with calcium as a biological team. Again, the problem is not the amount of calcium we take in, at all, but rather the ABSORPTION of it. As mentioned before, we generally don't get enough magnesium, boron, strontium, or vitamin D to help calcium be absorbed and to grow new bone cells.

Should we take calcium supplements? Are there benefits to adding calcium to the food we eat? Yes. Studies show that supplementation helps to slightly lower blood pressure, is good for our heart and artery health, can alleviate some symptoms of PMS, is necessary for brain metabolism, helps prevent intestinal tumors (colorectal adenomas), is necessary for blood clotting, and has many other uses other than making new bone cells.

# Chapter 4: Magnesium

Magnesium is number 12 on the Periodic Table, the seventh most abundant element, and was discovered in 1808. It has an atomic weight of only 24.3. It is one of the ten essential minerals with an RDA of 400 mg a day. It is the fourth most abundant mineral in our bodies, and fifth most in the oceans. While mammals use iron as the center of their blood molecules, plants use magnesium as the center of their chlorophyll molecules. Chlorophyll, of course, is the lifeblood of the plant world. Many soils are deficient in magnesium, as farmers rarely replace it when using commercial fertilizers that tend to facilitate leaching of minerals from the soil. Most people do not get sufficient intake of it with Americans generally taking in only about 300 mg, at best. Fortunately you can easily obtain an inexpensive supplement of 200 mg or more. Common salts such as citrates, lactates, or oxides are all bio-available.

Even the most nutrient-rich mineral water doesn't provide much magnesium. The American diet has been shown to be generally low, due to the extensive refining and processing of our foods, especially whole grains. The best dietary sources of magnesium are plant sources, especially whole grains, dried beans, and nuts, but the fact that Americans consume so few whole grains creates deficiencies. Black Americans have been shown to be especially low due to their ethnic diets, the elderly are showing an increased need exacerbating the many problems of aging and people of all economic levels are deficient. One-in-seven Americans has seriously low serum levels. Toxicity is not a concern. I recommend everyone consider a daily supplement, since my research conclusively shows magnesium to be beneficial. Because it is such a vital and essential nutrient, every year the studies performed on magnesium is over-whelming. Four hundred years ago people were eating Epsom salts (magnesium sulfate) as a cure-all, and but for the laxative effect, the nutritive benefits they received were not realized.

Magnesium is used in so many biological functions it is impossible to cover them all. It affects numerous processes and actually may be the most important of all minerals in human nutrition. New benefits for healthy magnesium levels are continually being discovered. Studies of the most common acute and chronic illnesses and conditions that affect us often show low serum levels. Deficiencies of magnesium may be the most under-diagnosed of all mineral shortages. Drinking coffee or alcohol, eating too much salt, drinking sodas (phosphoric acid), coping with the stress of modern life, and taking prescription drugs all help deplete what magnesium we do take in.

Cardiovascular health is one of the basic and important needs, and includes heart attacks, hypertension, strokes, athero-sclerosis (plaque buildup), high blood fats, and congestive heart failure. Study after study show that people with higher serum levels simply have less heart and coronary disease, lower blood pressure, fewer strokes, and lower cholesterol levels. Heart and artery conditions are *the* leading cause of death among Westerners, by far. Having a high serum magnesium level is a good way to help prevent CHD (coronary heart disease).

Illnesses such as Diabetes and insulin resistance are correlated with hypo-magnesium (low) levels. Oxidative stress is part of the diabetes syndrome and is shown to be magnesium-related. Any program that treats blood sugar disorders should include a magnesium supplement (minimum 200 mg per day). As we age, the bone loss we experience is partly due to magnesium deficiency. Bone mineral density depends on magnesium, boron, strontium, and vitamin D in order for calcium to make new bone cells. There is an important calcium-to-magnesium ratio—half as much magnesium as calcium should be in your supplement. As many as 40 percent of asthmatics have been shown to have low serum levels. Therefore, treatment of this condition should always include magnesium. Inexpensive supplementation has shown dramatic results from both migraine and muscle tension headaches. Women have found that magnesium can help alleviate some of the symptoms of PMS, which affects the great majority of American females.

This wonderful mineral is needed for hormone metabolism, neuromuscular function, energy metabolism and exercise performance, the prevention of various cancers, liver function, skin metabolism, vitamin metabolism, water balance in our bodies, over 300 known enzyme reactions. It is a basic mineral catalyst to accelerate countless biological reactions

# Chapter 5: Iron

The fourth most abundant element, Iron is number 26 on the Periodic Table, and has been known to man since the beginning of time. It has an atomic weight of 55.8 and is, therefore, a heavy metal. The research on iron is very extensive, partly because three-fourths of it is the "heme" in hemoglobin, or red blood cells. Iron makes blood red and transports oxygen from our lungs. This is one of the ten minerals with an established RDA—10mg for men and 18mg for women. Most all vitamin/mineral supplements have iron in them as common sulfates, fumarates, and gluconates. Children, pregnant women, and often older people, have higher needs for iron. A good supply of iron is found in most any seafood, meat, poultry or organ food like liver, and also in many vegetables such as beans and peas, nuts, seeds, and green vegetables.

The body only absorbs iron as it is needed and simply excretes the excess. Sufficient copper in the body is needed for its proper absorption. There is an important iron-to-copper relationship in mammals. Recently media attention has been given to the people who have too much iron and require "iron free" vitamin- mineral supplements. One contributing factor is that these people nearly always take in far too much iron from meat, poultry and other animal foods. The real problem is that they have an *absorption* malfunction whereby they store iron they don't need.

Reports consistently reveal that most Americans, especially women and vegetarians, simply don't get enough iron in their diets. Deficiencies can manifest as anemia, weak blood function, heartburn, dizziness, headaches, sore tongue, hair loss, digestive problems, nausea, sensitivity to cold, irritability and loss of appetite. Older people often respond well to iron supplements, with more energy and endurance even though they show no evidence of iron deficiency. While the main use for iron is by the red blood cells, every cell in our bodies contains it. It is necessary for support of our immunity, enzyme reactions, energy metabolism, muscle function, and many other uses. Make sure you add this to your supplement program.

# Chapter 6: Zinc

Number 30 on the Periodic Table is zinc. This element was discovered back in the 13$^{th}$ Century. It has an atomic weight of 65.4 and is considered a heavy metal. Our bodies contain about 2.5 grams and it is found throughout our entire system with half of it in our muscle tissue. For example, the male prostate gland contains ten times as much as other organs. The established RDA is 15 mg and most Westerners simply do not meet those levels. Especially at risk are alcoholics, the elderly and poor people. Zinc can easily be toxic and you should never take in more than about 50 mg a day. Excess quantities will cause negative side effects such as cholesterol dysmetabolism, low HDL cholesterol, low white cell blood count and gastrointestinal disturbances. Zinc is found in most vitamin mineral supplements as sulfate, citrate or oxide, and are inexpensive, bioavailable sources. Zinc has an important relationship with copper and with iron in mammals.

There is so much research on zinc during the last forty years it is pretty overwhelming. Zinc is one of the most studied of all minerals. It is found in whole wheat, brown rice, oats, lentils, soybeans, dried peas, black-eyed peas, lima beans, walnuts, peanuts, cashews, brazil nuts, many cheeses, any kind of liver, animal flesh such as beef, lamb, chicken, turkey, various fish and seafood.

Zinc is needed for the synthesis of RNA and DNA, growth and development, to fight inflammation, sexual maturity, reproduction, immunity, healing wounds, thyroid function, production of prostaglandins, blood clotting, development of the fetus, production of sperm, building bone cells, for over 100 body enzyme reactions, skin metabolism, good vision, our senses of taste and smell, and too many other processes to even try to list. Zinc (zinc oxide and zinc pyrithione creams or sprays) has powerful topical uses as well. Zinc deficiency is common in America, especially in children, but is very easy to remedy with a simple 15 mg supplement every day. Deficiencies include anemia, delayed growth in children, birth defects, spontaneous abortion, sterility, impaired sexual maturity, glucose intolerance and various bone conditions.

# Chapter 7: Boron

Boron is number 5 on the Periodic Table and was discovered in 1808. It has an atomic weight of only 10.8, making it the lightest of all essential minerals. No one now disputes how vital it is to plant and animal life, but it wasn't until 1990 that it was finally accepted as essential for humans. This is truly the most overlooked and neglected supplemental mineral even though the research on it is very extensive and Boron has been available for almost two decades with is no RDA established to date, but I feel a daily intake of 3 mg would be sufficient.

Due to modern farming methods, our soils are boron deficient. Therefore, you cannot rely on whole grains, beans, vegetables, and fruits to consistently supply this vital mineral. Sea vegetables may be the only reliable food source. Toxicity is rare, except in factory workers who are exposed to it. In areas where the crops and the soil are rich in this mineral, longer life spans and less morbidity (disease rates) are found. You would think that all vitamin and mineral supplements would contain a mere 3 mg of boron, but such is not the case. Take a look in the largest vitamin catalogs in the world and you will rarely even see boron in their top-of-the line premier formulas, much less in the 3 mg amount you need. One of the top three vitamin catalogs refuses to add it to any of their vitamin/ mineral formulas, and offers only 0.75 mg (one-fourth of what you need) in its boron-only product! It is vital to take a boron supplement, no matter how well you eat, because our daily food contains so little. Any reasonable salt including inexpensive boric acid is bioavailable. Some farmers do add boron salts to their soils, but this is not common practice at all. Few ranchers add boron to their livestock's feed.

The research on boron is overwhelming, yet most people are seriously deficient. Study after study shows that Americans only eat about 1 mg a day, with vegetarians getting the most. Boron is necessary to bone and cartilage metabolism and is beneficial to people suffering from arthritis or osteoporosis. Bone and cartilage metabolism may be the most important of all benefits, especially since arthritis and osteoporosis are becoming epidemic. Boron and other mineral deficiencies are one of the basic reasons for these conditions. In human research boron supplementation has been shown to help relieve arthritis and osteoporosis. Taking calcium, magnesium, strontium, and vitamin D along with it makes a powerful healing combination. Westerners take in more calcium than anyone else, but have the most bone and joint diseases, because the calcium cannot be *absorbed* without boron (along with magnesium and vitamin D). In general, boron is vital to hormone metabolism, and it is the only mineral supplement that can raise low sex hormone levels. For example, high boron supplements may actually raise testosterone levels, in both men and women. It is vital to reproduction and pregnancy, countless enzyme reactions, athletic performance, vitamin D metabolism, brain function and cognition, blood metabolism, immune function, and many other important health factors.

Boron has been shown to be an important factor in cardiovascular health with deficiencies contributing to hypertension (high blood pressure). Cholesterol levels and metabolism depend on boron as does hormone metabolism and especially our sex hormones. Athletes have shown better performance, while weightlifters and bodybuilders have achieved impressive results from taking boron. In our brains, boron levels show positive effects on cognition, memory and even mental diseases. Women given boron supplements got relief from PMS, as well as menopausal symptoms. This is important for women of all ages. Boron has been shown to be important in diabetes and insulin resistance Boron has been shown to be necessary in thyroid metabolism, and low thyroid activity is epidemic in Americans over the age of fifty. Laboratory animals given boron in their feed lived 10 percent longer than controls, with no other changes.

We are finding that a common factor in certain cancer rates is boron deficiency. More research is needed on the relationship between cancer and boron (along with other minerals) instead of allopathic (covering up the symptom while ignoring the cause) surgery, radiation and chemotherapy. Science has been clear on the vital need for adequate boron intake for over twenty years, but most of us still aren't taking a simple, inexpensive, safe 3 mg dose every day. For all the proven benefits and protection it provides, add this mineral to your daily supplement regime.

# Chapter 8: Manganese

Number 25 on the Periodic Table and discovered back in 1774. It has an atomic weight of 54.9. The research on manganese can be overwhelming in many aspects. Manganese is one of the ten minerals with an established RDA only recently set at 2 mg. Our bodies normally contain less than 20 mg obtained mostly from a diet of grains, beans, nuts, seeds, and green vegetables. Common vitamin and mineral supplements contain this as simple sulfates or oxides. Even though it is a heavy metal, manganese is not considered toxic, and people with illnesses can take up to ten times the RDA (i.e. 20 mg) without side effects.

Common dietary sources are whole grains such as wheat, rye, oats, brown rice, corn, various dried beans and peas, nuts and seeds, leafy greens, root vegetables such as sweet potatoes and beets, and, of course, sea vegetables. The refining of grains takes much of the manganese out of our diets. This is one of the minerals that scientific farmers put in their soils to insure good crops Ranchers often use manganese in the mineral supplements they give to livestock.

Manganese is necessary in our bodies for insulin production, fat metabolism, growth factors, reproduction, muscle coordination, neurotransmitter function, lipoprotein metabolism, our oxidation defense system, bone and cartilage growth, enzyme activity, proper blood clotting, oxidative stress and SOD function. Deficiencies result in such problems as bone and cartilage disease, some cases of deafness, carpal tunnel syndrome, repetitive motion syndrome, infertility and stillbirths, low libido, menopausal problems, and convulsions. Excessive manganese consumption is basically confined to factory workers at refineries and smelters.

Recently, research has shown the benefits of supplementation in arthritis and osteoporosis. This is due to the necessity of synthesizing mucopolysaccharides, which make up support and connective tissue, especially cartilage, tendons and bone cells. Other research has shown promise in such conditions as epilepsy and tardive dyskinesia.

# Chapter 9: Copper

Number 29 on the Periodic Table and discovered over 6,000 years ago. Copper has an atomic weight of 63.5 and is a heavy metal. It is one of the ten minerals with an established RDA, which is 2 mg. Our body only contains about 150 mg of this vital mineral. The research on copper is overwhelming and continuing. Copper levels vary in each individual. For example, one person with arthritis may have both high and low serum blood copper levels. Copper can be found in many vitamin/mineral supplements in the form of inexpensive copper salts (citrate, gluconate or cupric oxide), that are all very easily absorbed. Copper, like zinc, can be toxic. While it is rather difficult to take in excess, as little as 15 mg daily could cause such side effects as nausea, abdominal cramps, vomiting, and diarrhea.

The main reason people often have copper deficiencies is that their diets consist of refined whole foods especially whole grains. Ironically, poor people in Third World countries who do not refine their foods have little problem with such deficiencies. Many Americans only get about 1 mg per day in their food – half what they need. Some good dietary sources of copper include wheat, barley, sunflower seeds, almonds, pecans, walnuts, peanuts, cashews, prunes, raisins, apricots, various dried beans, mushrooms, chicken, and halibut. People whose homes contain copper plumbing that could leach the mineral into the drinking water should be getting more than enough copper, and highly acidic water could conceivably add to this

There is an important zinc-to-copper balance where these two metals interact and work together. For example, taking in too much zinc will interfere with copper absorption. Copper also helps us absorb iron and prevent anemia. Copper (and zinc) makes up the main form of superoxide dismutase (SOD), which is a basic anti-oxidant enzyme.

Copper is necessary for nerves, nerve transmission, many enzyme reactions, blood vessels, fighting inflammation, cholesterol levels, absorption of other minerals such as iron, and cardiovascular health in general. The uses for copper are simply far too numerous and complex to list.

14

# Chapter 10: Silicon

Silicon is number 14 on the Periodic Table and was discovered in 1824. It is the second-most common element on earth (making up 25 percent of the earth's crust), we still find deficiencies in our diets! It is very light, has an atomic weight of 28.0, and, like iodine, is not a metal. A good form is plain silica gel or silicic acid, which is both inexpensive and bio-available. Silicon is not to be confused with silicone—a polymer of silicon and oxygen—found in breast implants. By taking excess silica gel you may temporarily receive the unique benefit of absorbing excess aluminum in the body and excreting it (Americans tend to have high levels of aluminum in their blood). This is of great importance since excess aluminum is toxic and builds up in the brains of Alzheimer's patients.

There is no doubt at all that silicon is necessary to both plant and animal life, yet it still is not recognized by many scientists as a necessary mineral. In the last fifteen years there has been extensive research available on silicon, yet you do not see farmers or ranchers using it, or vitamins companies adding it to their formulas. Farmers should be adding such nutrients as inexpensive calcium silicate to their soils and should routinely feed supplements such as inexpensive silica gel to their livestock. We need more human studies as research is not nearly as extensive as it has been with agriculture or feed animals.

Animal research leaves no doubt as to the importance of silicon in our diets. Since it is not toxic, you can safely take 10 mg a day, which is a generous amount. It is difficult to figure out a daily value for it, as the amount in common foods varies so greatly. You will find silicon in fresh and frozen vegetables such as onions, beets, kale, tomatoes, cabbage, asparagus, cucumbers (technically these are fruits), and string beans, as well as brown rice, oats, lima beans and some fruits such as strawberries and peaches.

We do know silicon is necessary for bone and cartilage growth and anyone with arthritis or osteoporosis should be taking it. Silicon has received praise for its cardiovascular benefits. This is a mineral you need to add to your daily regime.

# Chapter 11: Iodine

Iodine is number 53 on the Periodic Table and was discovered in 1811. It has an atomic weight of 126.9 (the heaviest of the essential minerals) and is the only other essential mineral, besides silicon, that is non-metallic. It is a trace mineral and one of the ten with an established RDA (150 mcg), making it the only non-metallic mineral with a RDA.

A good source is potassium iodide, and you will find it in most vitamin/mineral supplements, as well as iodized table salt. Table salt has offered an iodized variety (avoid any added aluminum salts) for over 80 years now to combat goiter, which thankfully has almost disappeared. The best dietary source is seafood and sea vegetables (i.e. seaweeds), although Westerners rarely will eat sea vegetables. ). Some varieties, such as kelp, can be too high in iodine and may cause skin problems such as acne, eczema and dermatitis due to excess iodine intake. A mere teaspoon of kelp powder can contain 20 times the RDA. People who eat seafood even a few times a week need not worry about a deficiency. People who do not eat ocean fish and seafood should definitely take a supplement. Iodine in the soil varies so radically you cannot depend on grains, beans, vegetables, or fruits to supply it. Milk and dairy products have considerable iodine, but are a very poor dietary choice because they contain indigestible lactose.

Iodine is associated with the thyroid gland since that organ contains three fourths of the approximately 30 mg of iodine we have in our bodies. The other fourth is doing important work in our bodies, along with all the other minerals. Thyroid problems are almost never solved by iodine supplements, anyway, but rather require either T4 (L-thyroxine) and/or T3 (triiodothyronine). Both of these bioidentical hormones are iodine based, chemically.

Hypothyroidism (underactive thyroid) is very prevalent among Americans over fifty, while hyperthyroidism (overactive) is a much less common problem. It is very easy and inexpensive to get either a blood or saliva test for free T3 and free T4 to determine the status of your thyroid function. Low thyroid can have very dramatic effects on our health, metabolism and how much we weigh.

# Chapter 12: Chromium

Number 24 on the Periodic Table and was discovered back in 1797. It has an atomic weight of 52.0 and barely qualifies as a heavy metal that can be accumulated easily in the body. Chromium is a trace mineral with an established RDA of 120 mcg. Fortunately, many vitamin mineral supplements do contain it. Brewer's yeast is highly allergenic and not recommended as a source. People with blood sugar disorders can take 400 to 600 mcg, for the first year. The toxic level is very low, but it is also very difficult to get much chromium unless you work with the refining and manufacturing of it. Research abounds regarding the value of chromium, especially for diabetes, insulin resistance, and hypoglycemia.

Much of our soil has sufficient chromium, as do many farm animals, which are either fed whole grains or allowed to graze freely. Humans are generally deficient because of the refined foods they eat, especially refined grains. This is more proof that whole grains, especially organically grown ones, are a staple food.

The most dramatic benefit of chromium supplementation is blood-sugar metabolism. It helps to normalize both high and low blood glucose. Epidemic rates of people who have insulin resistance and diabetes are due in part to chromium deficiency. Other contributors include the more than 160 pounds per capita of various sugars that are consumed each year. This overload of sugars also helps deplete what chromium we do consume. High insulin levels contribute strongly to heart disease, and diabetics suffer two to three times the heart attack rate. Research has shown a continual and serious decline in serum blood-chromium levels in the last fifty years. Some estimates reliably guess that 90 percent of Americans are deficient. Use any good salt or chelate as your supplement.

Coronary heart health is a second major benefit of getting enough chromium every day, and chromium helps keep cholesterol and triglycerides normalized. The average American adult has a deadly average level of 240 total cholesterol level. CHD is *the* leading cause of death, by far, in America and blood sugar dysmetabolism an epidemic. Chromium supplements will go a long way toward helping prevent and cure both of these conditions.

# Chapter 13: Vanadium

This is number 23 on the Periodic Table and was discovered back in 1801. It has an atomic weight of 50.1 and is considered a heavy metal. It is an essential trace nutrient for both plants and animals.

It has been known for over 30 years that vanadium is an essential mineral for mammals, yet there still is no RDA established. The best estimate is that 100 mcg (0.1 mg) is sufficient although some companies put an irresponsible 10,000 mcg (10 mg) in their products. Vanadium poisoning is extremely rare and confined to specialists who work with the manufacturing and refining of it. Few commercial supplements contain any vanadium at all. Look at the biggest catalog companies and notice they rarely add vanadium to their vitamin/mineral formulas. Whole grains and seafood are good sources of vanadium, but due to our poor soils, deficiencies are very common. Vanadium chelates are good sources as are common salts such as vanadyl sulfate. Prepared foods may show higher levels of vanadium due to intense contact with stainless steel, but this would not be very bioavailable and thus of little use despite the technical analysis.

The animal and human studies on vanadium have been well established in the last ten years. Blood-sugar metabolism is the most dramatic medical finding, since it is involved with bone, tooth and cartilage repair and maintenance.

The epidemic of insulin resistance and diabetes is certainly due, in part, to vanadium deficiency. Human studies on diabetes and insulin sensitivity have been available for over a decade yet, diabetics are almost never advised to use vanadium supplements to treat their condition. Any program of curing these must include a supplement. Vanadium has proven anti-cancer and anti-tumor properties and should be a part of any cancer prevention or treatment program. Vanadium is crucial to good heart and artery function, and even has blood pressure-lowering properties. It is vital to cholesterol and blood lipid metabolism. Vanadium has much to do with bone growth, as well as cartilage and tooth health. Short-term research has used high amounts as much as 10,000 mcg (10 mg), but this is completely contraindicated in long-term use. Do not use more than 1,000 mcg (1 mg).

# Chapter 14: Molybdenum

Number 42 on the Periodic Table and was discovered in 1781. It has an atomic weight of 95.9 and is very heavy. The potential for toxicity is limited mostly to those who work in refining, smelting and manufacturing of alloys with molybdenum. This is a trace mineral with an established RDA of only 75 mcg, but other estimates go as high as 250 mcg. The research on molybdenum is extensive and goes back decades, but is more concerned with soils, plants, livestock and toxicity, rather than essentiality and therapeutic benefits to humans.

This is one of the very few minerals that often is added back into the soil, and can even be found in plant food used by the home gardener. Many modern farmers make sure they enrich their soil with molybdenum for better crop yields and superior plants Some progressive livestock ranchers also make sure they feed their animals a mineral supplement with molybdenum. Most vitamin and mineral supplements should have the needed 75 mcg. The average American, surprisingly, may get enough of this every day, but soils and foods vary so dramatically that it is good insurance to make sure your vitamin/mineral supplement contains it.

This is not very toxic for such a heavy metal, and you would have to take 20 to 40 times the RDA (up to 10 mg) to get side effects from it. While there is a great deal of research on molybdenum, there is very little on its deficiency in various diseases and conditions. It is vital for many enzyme reactions, including over 30 known redox (reduction-oxidation) ones as it functions as an electron carrier. Anti-cancer and anti-tumor properties were attributed to molybdenum over thirty years ago, and his should be a part of any cancer preventive or treatment program. It is vital for treating bone and joint diseases such as arthritis and osteoporosis and it plays an important role in blood-sugar metabolism as well and should be included in your supplement program. Over forty years ago, it was shown to help alleviate iron deficiency anemia, and thirty years ago it was discovered that in lab animals it became an immunity enhancer. People with Wilson's Disease also have reported benefits from molybdenum supplementation. Since it is so safe this should included in your vitamin/mineral formula.

# Chapter 15: Selenium

Number 34 on the Periodic Table and was discovered back in 1817. It has an atomic weight of 79.0. It is one of the ten minerals with an established RDA, which is only 70 mcg. The RDA was only recently established, and selenium previously was considered toxic, rather than essential. I recommend not exceeding more than 200 mcg along with 400 IU of mixed tocopherol vitamin E as a synergist for even better results. Chelates are a good choice. The best food sources are whole grains, seafood, and, of course, sea vegetables. This is just one more reason to eat whole grains at every meal. Fortunately, you will find this in most vitamin and mineral supplements.

This is a very powerful antioxidant and is considered a "catalyst" element that accelerates other reactions. Most of our soils contain adequate levels of selenium, and livestock generally get enough selenium in their food, even though farmers rarely test their soils or add selenium supplements to the feed. Levels therefore vary greatly in various foods. It is the *processing* of such basic foods as whole grains that has led to widespread deficiencies. The symptoms of such deficiency are so wide ranging that they just cannot be named individually. This is a very powerful antioxidant and scavenges harmful free-radicals.

Selenium can be a very toxic mineral, and even as little as 1,000 mcg (1 mg) or less per day can result in serious poisoning. This is why it was considered toxic and why you must not take in too much. The most dramatic benefit of having healthy selenium levels is cancer protection, especially for such cancers as colon, prostate and breast. A comparison of 27 different countries showed that the higher the selenium intake the lower the cancer rates generally. Another major benefit is cardiovascular health. Another advantage is protection against diabetes and insulin resistance.

Some countries, like New Zealand and Finland, have selenium poor soils and get an average daily intake of less than 30 mcg. Research in Finland compared 12,000 people, and the ones with the lowest serum selenium levels had six times the cancer rate of those with the highest levels. Other Finnish research showed those with the lowest selenium levels had seven times the CHD conditions as those with the highest levels.

# Chapter 16: Germanium

Number 32 on the Periodic Table and was discovered in 1886. It has an atomic weight of 72.6 and is a heavy metal. Many scientists now generally recognize that germanium is a necessary ultra-trace mineral for both plant and animal life. It will soon be firmly established as necessary for human health. No RDA has been established for it but an adequate, yet not excessive dose would be 100 mcg a day. Germanium sesquioxide is safe and non-toxic, but germanium dioxide is toxic. Very irresponsible promoters were, and still are, selling germanium supplements with 100 mg of germanium. This is ONE THOUSAND TIMES more than you need—a three-year supply per day! On the other hand, you find equally unscrupulous promoters selling germanium with only a few biologically useless micrograms per dose. This mineral is not normally found in vitamin and mineral supplements.

Unfortunately, there is not a lot of research being done on germanium. We do know that it is contained in the soil, is taken up in plants, is present in animals and is found in humans. What little human and animal research that exists is very —within the last ten years—with the most promising coming out of China. More human studies are needed to compare levels of germanium in people with various diseases versus healthy controls. Antitumor and anticancer effects were found in laboratory animals. Chinese hepatitis patients at Potou People's Hospital were given germanium supplements, with good results. We will find out just how important germanium is, in the near future. We are already finding out how germanium helps keep our immune system strong. Research in both animals and humans is showing germanium deficiency exists in various cancers.

In 1988 a very impressive review was published in the Journal Medical Hypothesis, complete with 72 references. This was very convincing as to the benefits for the potential in enhanced immunity, oxygen enrichment of cells, free radical antioxidant scavenging, arthritis, osteoporosis, and anti-viral properties. We need more such work done for this very promising and important mineral.

# Chapter 17: Strontium

Strontium is number 38 on the Periodic Table and was discovered back in 1790. It has an atomic weight of 87.6. There is no doubt that strontium is an absolutely essential ultra-trace mineral for mammals based on the current research. Since vegetables and fruits vary so radically in content, the only foods that have consistent strontium levels are seafood and sea vegetables. It is very difficult to find a supplement containing any meaningful amount. Either an amino acid chelate or asparate is a good choice of form. Based on what is found in soils and various common foods, a reasonable estimate for a human adult dosage would be 1000 mcg (1 mg) daily. This would provide the needed amount without any possible toxicity.

Toxicity from strontium is almost unknown, since it is so hard to find in any quantity in soils or foods. (This has nothing at all to do with radioactive strontium-90, which does not exist in nature.)

Quite a bit of research has been done regarding the value of strontium to soil, plants, animals, and recently to humans. Yet, you do not see farmers adding it to their soil or giving it to their livestock, doctors using it in their practices, or even vitamin and pharmaceutical companies adding it to their formulations.

One of the most important functions found for strontium is in bone, teeth and cartilage metabolism. Arthritis, osteoporosis, dental caries (cavities), and other bone and joint diseases are epidemic in Western societies. We know that calcium cannot be absorbed without magnesium, boron and vitamin D. Now, we see strontium is another important factor in this. Instead of treating these conditions with toxic drugs, we should be using minerals and other natural supplements like glucosamine. Improved bone metabolism is only one of many benefits we are finding for having healthy strontium levels. Various diseases and conditions are being linked to a lack of strontium. For example, recent research found cytoprotective effects on the liver, which could help prevent cancer, cirrhosis and other liver diseases. Other research on animals and humans, have found low strontium indicated in various other types of cancer. Make sure a strontium supplement is an integral part of your healing program.

# Chapter 18: Nickel

Nickel is number 28 on the Periodic Table and was discovered back in 1751. It has an atomic weight of 58.7 and is a heavy metal. Nickel has been accepted as an essential ultratrace nutrient in plants and animals in very small amounts. It is vital for plant growth, especially the common foods we eat. The fact it is found in significant amounts in agricultural crops logically shows it is needed in human nutrition. A reasonable dose would be 100 mcg based on analysis of what is contained in diets of various cultures. Germans, Austrians and Indians, for example, were found to be eating about 80 to 130 mcg daily. Many people may not need a supplement, but taking 100 mcg is good insurance, since it varies so radically in different areas of the world. But, despite this fact, you will almost never find meaningful amounts of nickel in vitamin/mineral supplements.

Surprisingly, there is very extensive research on nickel in soils, plants and even some in animals, but hardly any in humans. At the University of Munich, the U.S. Department of Agriculture, and at Technische University, rats on a nickel-deficient diet developed health problems, especially with the liver, thyroid and folic acid and iron metabolism. We need more research on humans to see what benefits there are and what effects deficiencies cause. The few studies we have are far more concerned with toxicity than benefits. The University of Arkansas published an impressive review, with an impressive 109 references, on the need for dietary nickel and its effect on immunity. Nickel from manufacturing can build up in a few industrial areas and pollute their waters and soils. This excess nickel can then accumulate in plants. It is ironic this can happen, when parts of the world are deficient in it.

The few human studies have shown some very promising things about nickel. Chinese children with very high IQ's were much higher in serum nickel than normal children. Infertile women were shown to be very low in nickel, compared with fertile women of the same age. Nickel blood levels in diabetics have been shown to be lower than those of healthy controls. Pregnant women with low nickel levels suffered hypertension more often. Fertility is involved with nickel and other ultra-trace elements, and these serum elements vary in women during their monthly cycle.

# Chapter 19: Tin

Tin is number 50 on the Periodic Table and was discovered thousands of years ago. It has an atomic weight of 118.7 and is the second heaviest essential mineral after iodine. Based on studies of plant and dietary contents, 100 mcg of this ultra-trace mineral would be a reasonable daily intake. There is a fair amount of research on tin, but unfortunately most of it is on pollution from industry, rather than on its benefits for plants and animals. There are few human studies, and most of these are simply concerned with how much people take in from their food. There is no doubt this is essential, yet so little is known about it. We need more human research on this. It is almost impossible to find meaningful amounts of tin in any vitamin/mineral supplement. By the way, "tin cans" is a misnomer. Cans for food are not made of tin nor lined with tin, so they are not a dietary source because of leaching.

A complete search of the internationally published clinical studies did reveal a few very important findings that show how essential tin is. The problem is that tin is such a very heavy metal, and so prevalent from industrial manufacturing, that some areas are polluted that people get excessive tin in their blood, which is slowly excreted. Most of the research, therefore, is concerned with toxicity and pollution, rather than the necessity and benefits.

A series of antitumor drugs, called "organotin compounds" are based on the tin molecule and have shown good promise. The best of these studies was a review done at the University of Shizuoka, with an impressive 166 references. Tin is known to be involved in a wide variety of mammalian biological processes. The immune function generally depends on having sufficient tin. At Kyoto University in Japan it was clearly established that tin is essential in the diets of laboratory animals, determined by first feeding them both insufficient and then excessive amounts. At the University of Aberdeen, rare human research was done where serum tin levels were measured. These were compared to coronary heart health. It was found that low tin levels correlated with high LDL and n-6 fatty acid levels, both of which are predictors of CHD, in general. At the University of Medical Science (China), researchers did more human research, this time on peptic ulcers and gastritis, and found low tin levels.

# Chapter 20: Cobalt

Cobalt is number 27 on the Periodic Table and was discovered back in 1735. It has an atomic weight of 58.9. It is definitely an essential ultra-trace mineral for the simple reason that vitamin B-12 is based on the cobalt molecule. This is not the only use for cobalt at all, but simply the most important of them. We are said to synthesize our own vitamin B-12, but this would be impossible without sufficient dietary cobalt. The RDA for vitamin B-12 is only 6 mcg. A reasonable estimate for a dietary cobalt supplement based on content found in common foods grown in rich soil would be 10 mcg. Cobalt cannot be stored in the body, and therefore cannot accumulate. It is nontoxic and you would need over 100 times your daily need to possibly get any side-effects. There are a few areas in the world where cobalt from industry builds up in soil and crops, but this is rare.

The research on cobalt is very extensive, yet the world has simply not taken advantage of this research. Cobalt needs to be added to soil to yield better crops, because it is necessary to the plants for their optimum growth. Farmers need to give their animals cobalt, as livestock need it in their feed to develop and reproduce. Yet, it is basically impossible to find any vitamin mineral supplement on the face of the earth that contains cobalt, even though for decades science has known this to be essential in human nutrition. It is so easy and inexpensive to make sure our soils, our crops, our livestock, and real people get cobalt. So, why limit the use of cobalt to the synthesis of vitamin B-12? Cobalt has many other uses in our bodies, as we will find as we study it more.

Why not just take B-12 supplements instead of cobalt supplements? B-12 is only 4 percent cobalt, and we need it for many other processes. B-12 is absorbed extremely poorly when taken orally and the effective nasal sprays have not yet been approved by the FDA. Injections are expensive, invasive, and unpleasant.

For a complete nutritional supplement progressive pharmaceutical and vitamin companies will have to start adding this to their vitamin/mineral formulations. We are going to find more benefits for cobalt supplementation as the research continues.

# Chapter 21: Minerals We Might Need

It is interesting that there are only 13 vitamins, and that there is an established RDA for every one of them. We understand vitamins very well and that you can get a complete vitamin supplement inexpensively at any drug store. However, vitamins alone, have no value without the corresponding minerals that also naturally occur with them when in food. We still don't understand minerals very well, especially the ultra-trace elements that may only be needed in small, microgram amounts.

If you do a sophisticated analysis of sea water you will find most every known mineral, even if only in the smallest of detectable amounts. If you do the same sophisticated analysis of the various farming soils around the world you will also find most every mineral, even if only in barely analyzable amounts. You will also find an amazing variety of minerals if you analyze the common foods we eat, in the various countries of the world. Finally, if you analyze the human body you will still find most every known mineral contained in it.

Most importantly, when you analyze actual human blood you will find such varied elements as aluminum(!), antimony, arsenic(!), barium, beryllium, bismuth, bromine, cadmium(!), cesium, cerium, dysprosium, erbium, europium, gallium, gandolium, gold, hafnium, holmium, indium, iridium, lanthanum, lead(!), lutecium, mercury(!), niobium, neodymium, osmium, palladium, praseodymium, platinum, radium(!), rubidium, rhenium, rhodium, ruthenium, scandium, samarium, silver, tantalum, tellurium, terbium, thulium, thallium(!), titanium, tungsten, uranium(!), yttrium, ytterbium and zirconium.

These are the very same elements you find in similar amounts in seawater proving that the sea is the "mother of all life" and our blood a microcosm of the ocean. This is the reason sea vegetables are the best source of food minerals, with fish and seafood the second best source.

Which of these is necessary for plant life or for animal life? Which of these are actually necessary for us humans? Which ones are needed in nutrition, and which are poisons? Do we really need such elements as aluminum (the third most abundant element on earth), arsenic, cadmium, lead, mercury, radium, thallium and uranium which we consider poisons? Titanium is the ninth most abundant element on earth, yet currently shows no proof of being needed in plant or animal growth. We simply don't know at this point. Just because they exist in the oceans, in our soils, in plants, and even in our blood, does not necessarily mean they are essential for life. Some of these surely are toxic to us. Some of them are essential, but we haven't yet discovered which ones.

With the great advances in analytical technology we can now accurately detect minerals in our soils, the foods we eat, and our bodies. For the last decade, researchers around the world have been researching which ultra-trace elements may be essential. Which of these is the most promising?

*Cesium* may be the most promising of all, and has been studied quite a bit. International research shows benefits to animals, and indicates the same benefits when levels are measured in humans. *Rubidium* also has a surprising amount of research to show it is essential. In 1977 at both Schiller University (Germany) and Kyoto University (Japan), it was declared to be essential for plants and animals. *Barium* also has volumes of research behind plant and animal metabolism, thus providing evidence it is essential, (especially since we already take in about 1,000 mcg per day.) *Europium* has been shown to extend lifespan in test animals, and more research will be forthcoming. *Gallium* may well be essential, as it has been shown to be involved in bone metabolism. *Indium* is claimed to be beneficial on Internet promotions, but so far there is little to validate it. Surprisingly, *lanthanum* has had considerable research done on it and soon may well be shown to be essential. *Lithium* is definitely essential, but there doesn't seem to be a deficiency of it. The "therapy" of giving people with bipolar disorders 1,000 times the needed amount causes far more problems than it cures. *Neodymium* has potential in both human and animal health. *Praseodymium* has been studied revealing benefits to animals and humans. In plant and crop studies, *Samarium* also has shown potential as a nutrient, *thulium* (not to be confused with thallium) has a scarcity of research, yet a few soil and plant studies may indicate it may be classified as a necessary mineral. Lastly, *yttrium* may also turn out to be essential although there just isn't enough known about it so far. Only future research will answer these questions.

# RDA or Recommendation for mineral supplementation

| Mineral | RDA | Recommendation |
| --- | --- | --- |
| Calcium | 1000 mg | |
| Magnesium | 400 mg | |
| Iron | 10 mg men | |
| | 18 mg women | |
| Zinc | 15 mg | |
| Boron | 0 | 3 mg |
| Manganese | 2 mg | |
| Copper | 2 mg | |
| Silicon | | 10 mg |
| Iodine | 150 mcg | |
| Chromium | 120 mcg | |
| Vanadium | 0 | 100 mcg |
| Molybdenum | 75 mcg | |
| Selenium | 70 mcg | |
| Germanium | 0 | 100 mcg |
| Strontium | 0 | 1000 mcg |
| Nickel | 0 | 100 mcg |
| Tin | 0 | 100 mcg |
| Cobalt | 0 | 10 mcg |

# References

-J. Toxicol. Environ. Health (2001) v. 4, p. 395-429
-Baiquien Yike Daxue Xuebao (1999) v. 25, p. 373-4
-Guangdong Weil. Yuansu Kexue (1996) v. 3, p. 34-8
-Guangdong Weil. Yuansu Kexue (1996) v. 3, p. 51-5
-Guangdong Weil. Yuansu Kexue (1996) v. 3, p. 18-20
-Guangdong Weil. Yuansu Kexue (1999) v. 6, p. 22-8
-Guangdong Weil. Yuansu Kexue (1999) v. 6, p. 21-4
-Biol. Trace Element Res. (1998) v. 65, p. 45-51
-Biol. Trace Element Res. (1999) v. 68, p. 121-35
-J. AOAC Inter. (2001) v. 84, p. 1202-8
-Zhong. Fang. Yixue Yu Zazhi (2000) v. 20, p. 378-84
-Comm. Soil Science and Analysis (1999) v. 30, p. 2409-18
-Nutrition Res. (1998) v. 18, p. 11-24
-Biol. Trace Element Res. (1997) v. 57, p. 207-21
-Biol. Trace Element Res. (1997) v. 58, p. 91-102
-Biol. Trace Element Res. (1998) v. 59, p. 75-86
-J. Radio. and Nuclear Chem. (1997) v. 217, p. 139-45
-J. Radio. and Nuclear Chem. (1997) v. 222, p. 165-70
-J. Radio. and Nuclear Chem. (1998) v. 236, p. 123-31
-J. Radio. and Nuclear Chem. (1999) v. 239, p. 79-86
-Nova Acta Leopoldina (1998) v. 79, p. 157-90
-J. Commodity Sci. (2000) v. 39, p. 119-39
-Ciencia e Technol de Alimentos (2000) v. 20, p. 176-82
-Biotech. and Biotech. Equip. (2002) v. 16, p. 124-30
-Zhong. Gong. Weish. Xuebao (1998) v. 17, p. 104-5
-J. Toxicol. Environ. Health A (1998) v. 54   p. 593-611
-J. Toxicol. Environ. Health B(2001) v. 4, p. 395-429
-J. Agric. Food Chem. (1998) v. 46, p. 3146-9
-J. Agric. Food Chem. (1998) v. 46, p. 3139-45
-FASEB J. (1987) v. 1, p. 394-7
-J. Trace Element Exp. Med. (1992) v. 5, p. 237-46
-Food Addit. Contam. (1996) v. 13, p. 775-86
-Food Addit. Contam. (1998) v. 15, p. 775-81
-Food Addit. Contam. (1999) v. 16, p. 391-403
-Kidorui (1997) v. 31, p. 69-85
-Prac. Lek. (1997) v. 49, p. 68-78
-Sci. Total Environ. (1998) v. 216, p. 253-70
-Sci. Total Environ. (1998) v. 217, p. 27-36

-Sci. Total Environ. (1998) v. 218, p. 9-17
-Hokkaido Igaku Zasshi (1998) v. 73, p. 181-99
-Food Surveill. Paper (1998) v. 52, p. 1-113
-Crit. Rev. Food Sci. Nutr. (2001) v 41, p. 225-49
-Zhong. Huanjing Kexue (1997) v. 17, p. 63-6
-Hunan Nong. Daxue Xubao (1996) v. 22, p. 177-81
-Nippon Eiyo, Shok. Gakk. (1997) v. 50, p. 15-20
-Chem Letters (1997) p. 775-6
-Pathol. Oncol. Res. (1997) v. 3, p. 34-7
-Ann. Nutr. Metab. (1998) v. 42, p. 27-37
-J. Am. Diet. Assoc. (2001) v. 101, p. 294-301
-J. Food Compos. Analy. (1998) v. 11, p. 32-46
-Trace Element Elect. (1998) v. 15, p. 76-80
-Adv. Micronutrient Res. (1996) p. 19-44

# Other Books by Safe Goods

| | |
|---|---|
| *No More Horse Estrogen* | $ 6.95 US<br>$10.95 CAN |
| *The Natural Prostate Cure* | $ 6.95 US<br>$10.95 CAN |
| *Natural Born Fatburners* | $14.95US<br>$22.95CAN |
| *Lower Cholesterol without Drugs* | $ 6.95US<br>$10.95CAN |
| *Macrobiotics for Americans* | $ 7.95 US<br>$11.95 CAN |
| *Cancer Disarmed Expanded* | $ 6.95 US<br>$ 10.95 CAN |
| *What is Beta Glucan* | $ 4.95 US<br>$ 7.95 CAN |
| *Dr. Vagnini's Healthy Heart Plan* | $16.95 US<br>$24.95 CAN |
| *2012 Airborne Prophesy (fiction)* | $16.95 US<br>$24.95 CAN |
| *Spirit and Creator: The Mysterious Man Behind Lindbergh's Flight to Paris* | $39.95 US<br>$59.95 CAN |

*For a complete listing of books visit our website*
*www.safegoodspub.com*
*Order or call for a free catalog (888) 628-8731*